THE NEW JUICING FOR CANCER RECIPES BOOK

Ultimate Guide To Nutricious And Cancer Fighting Recipes To Build Your Immune System.

By

DONNA MARKS (RDN)

Introduction

Juicing is a terrific technique to increase the number of servings of fruits and vegetables in a diet that already contains plenty of them. Juicing is the act of separating the juice from the pulp of fruits, vegetables, and plant foods.

Juicing greatly reduces the amount of fiber you get from a vegetable or fruit; thus, it shouldn't be utilized to satisfy basic nutritional demands. This is valid for those who are in good health, can chew and digest their meals regularly, and aren't unintentionally losing weight.

Juicing may be a useful alternative for ensuring that your body receives essential nutrients if you are undergoing active treatment, have chewing, swallowing, or digestive issues, struggle with excessive weight loss as a result of cancer and its therapy, or have any of these conditions.

You might also want to think about blending your fruits and veggies to create nutritious "smoothies. " Consult a certified dietitian for advice on how to do this safely if you have trouble swallowing and to make sure you get all the calories and protein you need.

Juicing to increase your consumption of colorful fruits and veggies might be a healthy choice if you already consume five or more servings of these foods each day. For information: Half a cup of chopped veggies or fruit constitutes one serving.

If you aren't already getting your five servings of fruits and vegetables each day, start by doing this. Your first five portions should be made up of whole foods rather than juice. You can start juicing once you make it a habit to eat five servings of fruits and vegetables every day.

Include more veggies than fruits in your juices for the healthiest results. Make the remaining ingredients veggies since they have fewer calories and will make for a healthier drink overall. Add one fruit to your mixture to sweeten it. Juice one carrot, a slice of cucumber, a small beet, some ginger, and a small apple, for instance.

Juice has more calories and nutrition per unit of volume than entire foods. For instance, four to six large carrots are required to produce eight ounces of carrot juice. The majority of people wouldn't consume this many carrots at once. Juice in moderation to avoid consuming too many calories, which can lead to weight gain.

Include a dish of protein and a small amount of fat in your juice. Protein counteracts the juice's carbohydrate content, while fat facilitates your body's absorption of the juice's fat-soluble elements. For instance, if you juice first thing in the morning, pair it with some Greek yogurt and top it with some nuts and seeds.

Alternatively, pair your juice with boiling or scrambled eggs.
Use your imagination when juicing to prevent consuming too much of a few particular nutrients. You obtain the widest variety of nutrients by mixing them up. Even objects that you might normally discard, like broccoli stems, can be juiced. tally the crucifers. Broccoli, kale, chard, bok choy, kohlrabi, Brussels sprouts, cauliflower, watercress, collard and mustard greens, turnips, radish, daikon root, and arugula are examples of cruciferous vegetables.

These meals promote our body's natural detoxification processes, yet even healthy foods can be harmful to our health if consumed in excess. Consuming one to two servings of cruciferous vegetables daily is associated with no negative effects and a lower risk of several forms of cancer. Again, embrace variation! When a food is prepared differently, you absorb different nutrients from it in the same way that you acquire different nutrients from other foods.

The nutrients you take in from a cooked carrot differ from those from a raw carrot, which differ from

those taken in from carrot juice. You risk missing out on important nutrition if you only juice a portion of each serving of a certain dish. Always put food first. Once you've reached your daily target of five whole fruits and vegetables, try juicing to give your already healthy diet a boost.
Perhaps you've heard that juicing prevents cancer.

Antioxidants can be found in abundance in both fruits and vegetables. Cancer is combated by antioxidants. This may be the reason why some individuals think an "all-juice" diet can help with cancer treatment or prevention. While there are various health advantages to juicing, an "all juice" diet is not advised for those who have cancer or are receiving cancer treatment.
Always keep in mind that while juicing is a terrific way to include more fruits and vegetables in your diet, you shouldn't try to use it as a substitute for a balanced diet.

CHAPTER 1: Understanding Nutritional Needs.

Nutrition may not be the first thing that comes to mind when you consider fighting cancer. Healthy eating is emphasized in cancer prevention programs as a way to reduce your risk of getting the disease. What happens, however, after a cancer diagnosis? Do good nutrition and diet matter?

After receiving a cancer diagnosis, patients or their loved ones frequently begin to consider how food may impact the disease and the course of treatment. Your well-meaning friends may give you advice on what diet to follow, what foods to avoid eating, and how to incorporate different herbs and nutritional supplements into your diet. You can look for information online, but it may be overwhelming, contradictory, and perplexing. It's difficult to know who to believe.

Patients Frequently Ask The Following Wuestions:

Do I have to consume only organic or non-GMO foods?

Consider a ketogenic diet. Would that be useful?

Must I become vegan?

Do I need to take any dietary supplements?

Can sugar cause cancer?

Although these are valid concerns, the major objective of eating throughout cancer treatment should be to maintain your capacity to endure therapy and become ready for survivorship. Many patients are unaware of their risk for malnutrition or dehydration, and they aren't aware that these problems can make it more difficult for them to finish their treatment. In reality, many patients have major concerns about undernourishment, which refers to not getting enough food or nutritious nutrients. It's a frequent consequence of some cancer treatments and their associated negative effects.

On the other side, overeating (consuming more food than is necessary) also causes issues.

In addition to having a negative effect on therapy, obesity as a risk factor has been linked to decreased survival rates for several cancers, such as breast and prostate cancer. It may occasionally also result in a higher risk of cancer development or recurrence.

Getting the proper kinds of nutrients in the right amounts is the goal of good nutrition for cancer patients, which includes competing goals of quantity and quality. This article will cover the following to assist you with your diet throughout cancer treatment:
what to eat when receiving cancer therapy.

Dehydration and malnutrition are common causes, as are warning signals that you may require nutritional support. Where to obtain nutrition assistance for cancer patients.

How friends and family can support you: Call us or start a live chat online with a member of our staff if you have any questions about nutritional assistance during cancer treatment or holistic approach to cancer care at Cancer Treatment Centers of America® (CTCA).

Why is healthy eating critical during cancer treatment?

Maintaining a healthy weight, muscle mass, and energy levels before and after treatment depends on getting enough nutrition. This can help you tolerate therapy better and lower your risk of experiencing negative side effects.

The American Cancer Society states that eating well while undergoing treatment helps your immune system, which may reduce your chance of infection and hasten your healing and recovery. Fatigue and a decreased quality of life while undergoing treatment are frequently caused by nutritional deficits.

People who have long struggled with their weight may start losing a few pounds throughout treatment and not consider it to be a serious issue. However, even slight weight loss may increase your risk of adverse medication effects and possibly require adjusting or stopping your treatment. When hospitalization is required, severe malnutrition or dehydration may cause hospitalization and/or longer hospital stays.

Energy for exercise: If you lose weight while receiving treatment, it's possible that you're losing muscle mass and strength rather than fat that has been stored.

Maintaining your weight and energy levels through a healthy diet might provide you with the endurance to continue being physically active and carrying out your daily tasks. The American Society of Clinical Oncology offers several other potential advantages of exercise during and after therapy, as well as guidelines for safe exercise during treatment, **including:**

- Reducing the possibility of negative effects from the treatment lowering the risk of anxiety and sadness.
- Enhancing the quality of sleeplowering the danger of contracting more malignancies and other chronic disorders.
- Try to mix in some resistance training and cardiovascular activity as much as you can.

Exercises for breathing, balancing, and stretching may also be beneficial.

protection of the immune system. The immune system may become damaged during cancer treatment. In addition to targeting cancer cells, chemotherapy can also target healthy cells. Surgery may put a strain on the immune system as the body works to repair surgical wounds and avoid infection.

Furthermore, despite recent improvements in radiation therapy's accuracy, some healthy cells may still be damaged by the procedure. Some medical procedures can also result in situations that reduce the generation of white blood cells, which weakens the body's defenses against infection. There's a significant probability that being undernourished, especially if you're not getting enough calories or protein to keep your weight stable, is having a bad effect on your immune system.

Getting ready for survival: The advantages of adopting a healthier diet and exercise routine while receiving treatment may extend to survivorship. According to the National Cancer Institute, studies show that these healthier habits may increase certain cancer survivors' quality and duration of life.

Implementing the American Institute for Cancer Research's 10 Cancer Prevention Recommendations, which call for keeping a healthy body weight, obtaining enough exercise, and adhering to other dietary recommendations, is advised for cancer survivors. By following these recommendations, you may also lower your risk of obesity, which has been linked to a higher chance of acquiring 13 different cancers and a recurrence of some malignancies, including breast cancer.

You may be able to control or avoid other chronic conditions like diabetes or heart disease with the aid of a better lifestyle.

What foodstuffs are recommended during cancer treatment?

The difficulty with nutrition during cancer treatment is finding the correct balance between quantity and quality of food and nutrients consumed, given your unique disease type, treatment, and potential adverse effects.

The general population's dietary recommendations apply to a healthy diet for cancer patients as well: a balanced, plant-forward diet with whole grains, lean protein sources, fruits, vegetables, and minerals.

Whole grains like buckwheat, quinoa, brown rice, and whole wheat1-2 cups of vegetables per day1-2 cups of fruit every day. Several times per week, eat skinless chicken and cold-water fish like salmon, tuna, and cod. Added protein from dried beans, peas, lentils, and legumes. Olive oil, avocado, almonds, and seeds are examples of good fats.

Low-fat dairy products or a calcium replacement: fresh waterRed meat, processed meats, refined carbs, and added sugar should all be consumed in moderation.
Don't worry if you occasionally consume meals that aren't regarded as healthy. The only thing that sounds nice is a hot dog or some ice cream, so that is acceptable.

To discuss your unique dietary requirements, consult your care team. Inquire with your medical team about any dietary advice that might be related to the type of cancer you have, your course of treatment, or any potential side effects. Limiting your intake of fiber, for instance, may be beneficial if you have a bowel obstruction. Patients may be recommended to change what they eat and take some oral nutrition supplements because chemotherapy has a significant risk of nausea and vomiting.

Patients frequently inquire about using supplements. Some supplements may be helpful in managing treatment side effects when used properly, but they shouldn't be used to make up for a bad diet. Some supplements might even be hazardous or result in symptoms that aren't normal.

Regard food safety with greater care while receiving cancer therapy. You might be immunocompromised, depending on your treatment. Your white blood cell or neutrophil count may be impacted by some therapies, which could increase your chance of contracting a foodborne infection.

Try to be vigilant about keeping up with standard kitchen safety precautions while undergoing treatment, such as heating and storing food at the appropriate temperatures and being careful to disinfect cutting boards and prevent cross-contamination.

Common Reasons Cancer Patients Experience Malnutrition And Dehydration.

Malnutrition and dehydration can occur in patients even when they are actively attempting to eat healthily and stay hydrated due to circumstances brought on by the cancer itself and treatment-related adverse effects. A patient's nutritional condition may be impacted by a number of more prevalent symptoms, including an absence of appetite, nausea, and swallowing issues.

Cancers Linked To An Oncreased Risk Of Malnutrition.

Cancer-related side effects may impair the body's capacity to consume, digest, absorb, and metabolize food.
Due to the accompanying challenges with eating, swallowing, and digestion, patients with gastrointestinal malignancies are more likely to have malnutrition.

These tumors consist of:

- Malignancies of the head and Neckstomach cancer.
- Belly cancer
- Stomach cancers.
- Cancer of the pancreas.
- Intestinal cancer

Additionally, typical among people with advanced lung cancer is malnutrition. Lung cancer treatments may result in gastrointestinal issues and metabolic changes, including the generation of cytokines, which can cause anorexia (a severe loss of appetite), as well as weight loss and/or muscle wasting. Patients with this illness who have lung cancer may benefit from a feeding tube or an appetite stimulant.

Adverse Effects Of Treatment That Could Lead To Malnutrition And Dehydration.

Malnutrition and dehydration are potential side effects of cancer treatment that include: Chemotherapy and radiation therapy are frequently accompanied by nausea and vomiting. According to the National Cancer Institute, these side effects might affect up to 80% of chemotherapy patients. Some malignancies, such as ovarian, pancreatic, stomach, and lung cancers, may be more likely to cause loss of appetite than others.

Additionally, some chemotherapy, radiation therapy, and immunotherapy treatments can cause it as a side effect. Mucositis comes from digestive tract inflammation, which frequently causes uncomfortable ulcers (also known as mouth sores) in the mouth, throat, and gastrointestinal tract. Particularly when treating head and neck cancer, chemotherapy or radiation therapy may have the unintended side effect of mucositis.

This negative effect can also be brought on by some immunotherapies and targeted medicines. Dry mouth can be a side effect of several chemotherapy drugs as well as radiation treatment for head and neck tumors. It can result in the salivary glands producing less saliva, which might alter the patient's sensation of taste and make swallowing challenging.

Damage to the taste buds brought on by chemotherapy, radiation therapy, and surgical oncology may lead to alterations in taste and odor. A decrease in appetite could be a result of these changes. Constipation and diarrhea are frequently side effects of chemotherapy, but they can also happen after surgery, radiation therapy, and some painkillers.

Cancer Patients' Dehydration.

Cancer patients who have the same side effects that cause malnutrition may also become dehydrated. Vomiting and/or diarrhea raise the obvious issue of dehydration, but inadequate eating and drinking can also be problematic.
Constipation, dry skin, headaches, and weariness are just a few signs of mild dehydration. Low blood pressure, a rapid heartbeat, a fever, loss of orientation, confusion, and shock can all result from severe dehydration.

Kidney stones and urinary tract infections can both be brought on by chronic dehydration.
If you're dehydrated, your therapy may need to be delayed or modified, and individuals who are severely dehydrated might need to be hospitalized. Severe dehydration left untreated could even be fatal.

Even if you don't believe you could become dehydrated during treatment, make an effort to stay hydrated.

Although it's generally advised to drink eight cups of water every day, how much you actually require depends on your body weight. (Divide your weight by two to get at that figure.) (How many cups you should consume each day is determined by multiplying the result by eight.)

Malnutrition And Dehydration Warning Symptoms.

Patients are routinely checked for indicators of malnutrition and dehydration, and these problems are attempted to be avoided by nutritional support services. It's crucial to be aware of the warning signs that could mean you need to get assistance if your care team is not keeping an eye on you.

These consist of:
- Loss of weight.
- Having trouble eating or drinking as you typically would.
- Difficulty swallowing or swallowing pain.

- A recent enlargement in your eyes or ankles.
- Constipation.
- Diarrhea.
- A drop in energy or level of activity.
- A cough that starts while you're eating and is more frequent if you have lung, head, or neck cancer.

If you are having any of these symptoms, speak with your care provider. There might be treatments available that can help. Additionally, supporting therapies like pain management, naturopathic support, cancer rehabilitation, and/or nutritional assistance may be helpful to you.

CHAPTER 2: Juicing Basics.

The most popular juices are fruit ones, and making them professionally demands careful attention to detail to guarantee a safe and hygienic final result. Juicing at high volumes calls for equipment beyond the basic home juicer.

Modern fruit juice production machinery is primarily imported from Sweden, America, Germany, and Italy. Japan enters the global market and grows quickly in the fruit juice equipment sector.

A fruit sorter, washer, elevator, pulping machine, crusher, juice extractor, concentrator, sterilizer, filler, etc. make up a full juice processing line. Various fruits require various production methods. Their types and purposes are as follows:

Equipment For Making Juice:

Common machinery used to produce fruit juices are as follows.

1. Fruit Elevator: Is used to connect two nearby methods and move fruits from a low to a high location. Usually positioned after the fruit sorter or in between the washer and the fruit sorter.

2. Fruit Washers: Divided into brush spray and fruit surfing washing machines. used for a rough and clean selection of fruits and vegetables, particularly carrots and other difficult-to-clean produce.

3. Fruit Crushers: Are divided into two categories: squirrel-cage crushers and hammer crushers. used as a primary fruit and vegetable crusher.

4. Preheat Machine: Used to preserve color, remove enzymes, and soften raw materials. Fruit pulping machine: used to pulp and extract juice or puree from kernel fruits, including kiwi, mango, peach, strawberry, apricot, tomato, and raspberry.

5. Fruit Pulping Devices, Juice extractor: consists of a belt and spiral juice extractor. applies to high-juice-yielding kernel fruits, such as apples, pears, and mangoes.

6. Vacuum Concentrator: Consists of an externally circulating fruit jam concentration apparatus and a juice-concentrating pan with climbing and falling films.

7. Tube-in-tube Pipe Sterilizer: works with medium- and low-viscosity raw materials; uses steam and hot and cold water as heat transfer agents.

8. Aseptic Filling Machine: Has an asepsis chamber attached. Finish the canning, measuring, sealing, and cover-opening procedures.

Features Of The Line That Processes Fruit Juice:

- The whole system comprises cleaning,
- elevating,
- sorting,
- crushing,
- juicing,
- preheating,
- enzymolysis,
- filtering,
- concentration,
- blending,

- degassing,
- homogenization,
- sterilizing,
- filling, and packing of fruit.

It also covers the entire process, from raw materials to packed products. pertains to the manufacturing of jam, concentrate juice, clear juice, and hazy juice.

Depending on how well it functions, the majority of these pieces of equipment can operate on their own or in conjunction with the juice processing facility. To save energy, the power supply can also be divided.

1 High technique: The machinery used to make fruit juice uses cutting-edge technology and premium materials, ensuring a scientific design, a small structural footprint, and a beautiful appearance.
Reasonable layout, self-contained software for each unit, and an organized pipeline are all designed to make presentation and operation easier.

2. Multiple functions: It can demonstrate the entire juice-making process and carry out the industrial manufacturing of fruit juice. In addition, it can be utilized to study sample testing, additive application, and juice processing formula research. juice production line.

3. Growing popularity of juice production machinery. High precision, high quality, and high speedThe machinery used in the manufacture of juice is getting more and more automated in order to handle large-scale production and improve economic efficiency. The ability to produce is greatly increased.

Multifunctional:

One piece of equipment with multiple uses. Several fruit varieties can be treated using the fruit pre-treatment device. In the interim, the milk, tea, and coffee sterilizing and filling machines function flawlessly.

In Mechatronics, The most significant development in juice production machinery is this. The controller system has embraced the programmable controller. Computer-controlled large-scale equipment is capable of intelligent adjustment and self-diagnosis.

Juice-only diets, such as those that involve vegetables and fruits, are known as juice cleanses. There might be a few documented advantages. But there are also a number of hazards associated with juice fasts.

Juices from fruits and vegetables are rich in nutrients and can be an important part of a well-balanced diet. Some people think that by ingesting these juices for a short while, the system can be "cleaned" and numerous health benefits can be obtained.

Important Facts Regarding Juice Fasts:

Juice cleanse proponents assert that it can aid in weight loss and help the body rid itself of toxins. Juice-based diets have not been shown to be beneficial by enough research. Liquid diets have been associated in research with a higher risk of eating disorders and major health consequences. During a juice cleanse, you typically only drink juice for a set amount of time. Juice-only diets typically end after less than two weeks. Some programs, though, might run longer.

Juice diets are risky, though, and one should only follow a liquid-only plan when under medical supervision.

The science behind juice cleanses will be covered in this essay.

Assistance is on hand. People with eating disorders and those who are close to them may experience significant reductions in quality of life.

The chance of recovery is significantly increased by early intervention and treatment.

The National Alliance for Eating Disorders provides a daytime helpline manned by qualified therapists and an online search engine for treatment alternatives for anyone who feels they or a loved one may have an eating disorder.

Dangers Associated With Juice Fasts.

Juice cleanses carry a number of hazards, according to the National Center for Complementary and Integrative Health.

Diets for cleansing typically include fewer calories. A lower caloric intake may cause you to temporarily lose weight, but this change is rarely permanent. A person may suffer symptoms of low blood sugar if they consume too few calories since their body will not have enough energy.

Fainting,
weakness,
dehydration,
headaches, and hunger are a few of these symptoms. A juice cleanser could not be getting enough fats or proteins in their diet. These are both essential for healing, bodily well-being, and cognitive function.

Malnutrition can result from the prolonged elimination of certain food categories. A person is more likely to become ill if they drink unpasteurized juices or juices that haven't undergone any further treatment to eliminate microorganisms. This is particularly true for elderly and extremely young individuals, as well as those with compromised immune systems.

A person may lose excessive amounts of nutrients in their stool during a juice cleanse if laxatives or other bowel stimulation techniques are used. Dehydration and an imbalance in electrolytes may result from this.

Pre-packaged juice cleanses that advertise big outcomes, like curing ailments or offering remarkable health advantages, should also be avoided. Typically, these assertions are not well supported by research.

Renal health Nutrient-rich fruits and vegetables are abundant and can support the kidneys' optimal function. Renal function may also benefit from increased fluid intake.
On the other hand, several foods contain large amounts of oxalate, a substance that, when ingested in large amounts, might raise a person's risk of kidney issues. Beets and spinach are among the foods high in oxalate.

Chronic kidney disease patients may be susceptible to oxalate nephropathy. Rarely, healthy individuals could also be vulnerable to this.
When the body is unable to eliminate enough oxalate through urine, it builds up in kidney tissue and causes oxalate nephropathy. Kidney failure may result from this in rare instances.

Benefits Of Juice Fasts

Juice cleanse proponents assert that their products can help people lose weight and detoxify their bodies of pollutants. Harmful compounds like artificial chemicals and pollution are known as toxins.
Weight loss Research has indicated that juice-based diets cause "physiologically harmful" weight reduction in those who follow them.

Additionally, developments in liquid diets have been linked to eating problems by researchers.
In a 2017 study, researchers gave twenty healthy individuals a three-day regimen of just six bottles of various juices each day. A variety of components, including greens, apples, cucumbers, lemon, cayenne pepper, and vanilla beans, were included in the juices.

The individuals dropped 3. 75 pounds (lb), or 1. 7 kg, on average, after the fast. Their weight was still, on average, 0. 91 kg (2. 01 lb) less during a 2-week follow-up. After the three days, the individuals did not report feeling better.

Juice cleanses may nevertheless result in temporary weight loss owing to calorie restriction, but once a person resumes a complete, balanced diet, they will ultimately induce overall weight gain (as per a 2017 review).
Changes in gut microbiotaA quick juice fast can change the amount of bacteria in a person's digestive tract.

Researchers discovered that the juice fast enhanced the numbers of Bacteroidetes, the bacteria linked to weight reduction, and decreased the amounts of Firmicutes, the bacteria linked to weight gain, in the same 2017 study.

The human body is capable of eliminating these compounds on its own, even if they can be harmful to health. A 2014 review found that there is not enough data to support the use of detoxification diets to remove toxins from the body.

Removal Of Toxins.

Juice cleanse proponents frequently assert that their regimens can aid in a person's systemic toxin removal.

Drinking more water helps improve kidney function, and some nutritional elements may aid in the body's elimination of non-organic waste. Juice cleanses and other detoxification diets do not, however, appear to have a detrimental effect on the removal of toxins due to a lack of data.

Eating a well-balanced diet and staying hydrated are the best ways to assist the body's natural cleansing processes.
How to carry out a juice fastJuice cleanses and other restricted liquid diets should only be followed under physician supervision.
Supporters of juice cleanses may suggest a variety of programs,

including:
consuming solely liquids and juices for a few days.
mixing juice consumption with nutritional supplements and colon.
"cleansing" techniques like enemas and colonic irrigation.
Juicing while following a particular diet to help with weight reduction.

Several juice blends that were utilized in the Scientific Reports investigation are as follows:

filtered water,
cayenne,
lemon,
almonds,
dates,
sea salt, and vanilla bean;
apple,
cucumber,
celery,
romaine lettuce,
lemon,
spinach,
kale, and parsley;
apple,
lemon,
ginger; and beet;
apple,
pineapple,
lemon, and mint.

A daily consumption of six of these juice combinations amounted to 1, 310 calories.

Options Not to Do a Juice CleanseJuice cleanses' effectiveness cannot be determined due to a lack of proof. The following options can be tried by someone who wants to assist their body's natural processes and reduce or maintain a healthy weight.

Intermittent fasting:

This is skipping meals for certain parts of the day while maintaining a regular diet during other times. Reviews have connected increases in insulin sensitivity and weight loss to intermittent fasting.

Balanced diet: The greatest strategies to maintain a healthy weight and aid in the body's detoxification process are to eat a balanced diet and drink enough water. diets based on plants: These diets, which are naturally high in fruits and vegetables and centered around minimally processed meals, have been linked to decreased body weight. A plant-based diet can, with careful planning, supply all the nutrients required for optimal health, perhaps reduce the risk of heart disease, and generally have a smaller environmental effect than diets that contain animal products.

Find out more about diets and nutrition here.
In briefIn the medical world, juice fasts are
contentious since they typically don't provide
long-term remedies for wellbeing or weight loss.
Instead, a healthy, well-balanced diet is what most
experts advise.

Anecdotal evidence is typically used to support the
potential health advantages of juicing. There seems
to be growing evidence that a juice fast may have
adverse effects on the body, such as lowering renal
function.
To safeguard their general health, people should
consult their doctor before beginning a juice fast to
determine whether their current juice regimen has to
be modified.

CHAPTER 3:
Immune-Boosting Juices.

It's time to start seriously boosting your immunity as the cold sets in and the wind starts to get through jackets! Freshly squeezed juices and natural smoothies are a terrific method to increase your vitamin and mineral consumption for boosting your immune system and, in the event that cold or flu symptoms do develop, for easing symptoms in addition to eating a healthy, seasonal, and fresh diet.

It is common knowledge that consuming a nutritious, well-balanced diet rich in fresh fruits and vegetables will enhance general health and wellbeing and supply vital vitamins and minerals to support immunity. However, drinking fruits and vegetables can also help increase immunity, as can eating them. As a matter of fact, some people would rather drink juice than consume the daily required allowance of fruits and vegetables because it's faster and simpler. Still, some juices are more potent than others when it comes to boosting your immune system.

Below Are Some Immunity Juice.

1. Kale Juice: Rich in vitamins A, C, and K, kale is a fantastic source of nutrition. Antioxidants, such as beta-carotene, which helps prevent diseases like heart disease, are particularly abundant in raw kale. Furthermore, studies have demonstrated that kale lowers LDL, or bad cholesterol.

2. Carrot Juice: Rich in potassium, vitamin A, and biotin, carrots are low in calories. They are brimming with carotenoids, which your body uses as potent antioxidants. These include lutein, beta-carotene, lycopene, and alpha-carotene. A reduced risk of heart disease, prostate cancer, and degenerative eye illnesses may be associated with carotenoids. Carrots make a great juice because of their mildly sweet flavor; they go well with beets or citrus.

3. Beet Juice: Rich in health benefits, earthy in flavor, and colorful, beets are a superfood. They are rich in nitrates, which may lower blood pressure and improve physical and mental performance. They are also loaded with manganese, potassium, and folate. When juicing, don't forget to include the beet greens—they're also full of nutrients!Orange Juice: Citrus fruits, including orange juice, are excellent providers of vitamin C. Antioxidants like vitamin C shield cells from things that harm the body.
Additionally, white blood cell and antibody production are enhanced by vitamin C, aiding in the body's defense against foreign invaders.

4. Tomato Juice: Rich in vitamins C and A, which are essential for a healthy immune system, tomato juice is a great source of these nutrients.

5. Kiwi Strawberry Juice with Mint: Mint is an herb that is high in folate, vitamin A, magnesium, and zinc, and kiwis and strawberries are both delicious fruits high in vitamin C. Kiwi strawberry juice combined with mint leaves the body feeling more resilient to illness.

Drinking Juice To Boost Immunity.

The juicing fad arose as a way to obtain the benefits of various fruits and vegetables in potent, blended beverages because it is feasible to reap the benefits of specific fruits and vegetables by ingesting them in juice form.
In addition to a nutritious diet and regular exercise, you can enhance your immune system and general well-being by following any of the thousands of juicing recipes available online.

These recipes combine the benefits of several fruits and vegetables to make a rich, immune-boosting smoothie or beverage. Tomato-carrot juice, for example, provides a potent antioxidant and vitamin A combination that enhances the health of collagen in the skin. It also acts as a barrier to entry for pathogens that might cause disease and controls the activity of immune cells, such as T-cells, B-cells, and cytokines. Not to mention, this combo works wonders for protecting your skin from the signs of aging.

Other combinations, like carrot-apple-pear juice, offer a pleasant and healthy substitute if you're not a huge fan of tomato juice. The options are endless: you can mix your own immune-boosting juices to boost immunity, combat the signs of aging, and fend off anything from the common cold to chronic disease once you've learned about the various immune-boosting effects of various fruits, vegetables, and even herbs.

CHAPTER 4:
Antioxidant-Rich Juices.

Since they have the ability to neutralize free radicals, stop oxidative damage, and fend off many chronic diseases, antioxidants are crucial for preserving your health. The best antioxidants that are vital to our well-being are astaxanthin, beta-carotene and lycopene, vitamins C and E, and phenolic substances including anthocyanins, quercetin, resveratrol, and catechins. Spirulina drinks, matcha, coffee, tea, dandelion tea, beet, pomegranate, acai, and lemon juices, green smoothies, and coconut water are some of the greatest liquids high in antioxidants.

Maintaining a well-balanced and nutrient-dense diet is crucial to maintaining optimal physical function. Furthermore, antioxidants are essential parts of every diet. They guard against sickness, preserve the integrity of our DNA, and keep our bodies healthy. Adding foods and beverages high in antioxidants to your diet is always a fantastic idea because doing so can have a number of health benefits, including the potential to prevent disease and slow down the aging process of your body.

Although most people know what foods are high in antioxidants in general, a lot of us also wish to add healthy antioxidant drinks to our diets to help them absorb more nutrients. We've compiled a comprehensive list of the top antioxidant-rich drinks in this book to keep you happy and healthy.

What is the purpose of antioxidant drinks?

A class of molecules known as antioxidants works to counteract free radicals, which are dangerous substances that damage DNA and cause cell deterioration. This can lessen inflammation, guard against chronic illnesses, and stop oxidative stress from harming the body's cells. Antioxidants can also boost the synthesis of antibodies and help prevent skeletal muscle damage brought on by oxidative stress during exercise.

All things considered, these substances are necessary for the survival of every living thing. Furthermore, obtaining antioxidants from food and beverages can only help you and your health, even if our bodies are capable of producing antioxidants on their own, such as the cellular antioxidant glutathione.

The Top 5 Antioxidants and Their Sources.

1. Carotenoids: Particularly lycopene and beta-carotene These antioxidants are present in watermelon, asparagus, tomatoes, apricots, carrots, pumpkin, kale, and cantaloupe.

2. Calcium E: Avocados, almonds, leafy greens, peanuts, red peppers, and sunflower seeds are good sources of this vitamin.

3. Vitamin C: Good sources of this antioxidant include bell peppers, Brussels sprouts, broccoli, cauliflower, grapefruit, oranges, sweet potatoes, and strawberries, in addition to leafy greens.

4. Astaxanthin: Eating more fish, seafood, and blue algae will increase your intake of this antioxidant. Particularly abundant in this nutrient are krill, salmon, and plankton.

5. Phenolic substances:
Resveratrol, which is present in wine, grapes, berries, and peanuts; anthocyanins, which are present in strawberries, blueberries, and tea; catechins, which are frequently found in tea, cocoa, and berries; and quercetin, which is abundant in

apples, red wine, and onions, are some of the antioxidants in this group.

Top Drinks for Antioxidants.

Although many health-conscious individuals attempt to increase the amount of antioxidants in their diet by consuming foods from particular food groups, beverages also contain a significant amount of antioxidants. In actuality, consuming just one or two antioxidant-rich drinks each day can significantly increase your nutrient intake and benefit many different bodily organs.

1. Spirulina-containing beverages: Spirulina is a form of filamentous cyanobacterium that has been added to food for centuries. Apart from its high protein and vitamin content, spirulina has numerous other possible health benefits. Its anti-inflammatory, immunomodulatory, and antioxidant qualities aid in the reduction of oxidative stress and the treatment of immune system problems. Consequently, this can aid in the prevention of numerous illnesses, including hypertension, heart failure, cardiac hypertrophy, and atherosclerosis.

Spirulina combats free radicals, increases the activity of superoxide dismutase and catalase, and activates the body's antioxidant enzymes. It also slows down lipid peroxidation and DNA damage. Furthermore, research has demonstrated that spirulina can increase the generation of antibodies and successfully protect skeletal muscle damage in situations where oxidative stress caused by exercise is present.
You can add spirulina powder to smoothies and drinks by dissolving it in hot water or tea.

2. Tea verde: Millions of people drink green tea, one of the most well-liked antioxidant beverages, every day all over the world. Epigallocatechin gallate (EGCG), a substance that has drawn a lot of interest and has been well researched for its antioxidant properties, is abundant in this beverage. This substance can strengthen your immune system, lower inflammation, and aid in weight loss. In addition, green tea has high concentrations of additional polyphenols and antioxidants, including epicatechin, gallic acid, and catechin.

3. Macha: Matcha tea is prepared by powdering entire tea leaves into a fine powder, adding hot water, and whisking the mixture with a bamboo brush until frothy. Since the entire tea plant is used to make matcha, it contains an exceptionally high concentration of antioxidants.

Matcha has been shown in certain studies to have numerous health advantages, such as preventing liver damage and slowing the growth of cancer cells. Furthermore, a 2017 study came to the conclusion that matcha may enhance memory, concentration, and reaction time.

4. Tea with Dandelion: The leaves and roots of the dandelion plant are brewed in hot water to create dandelion tea, a sort of herbal tea. Due to its ability to efficiently lower cholesterol, minimize oxidative stress, and reduce inflammation, dandelion has been extensively utilized in traditional medicine. Dandelion extract has been found to contain a significant amount of flavonoids, including luteolin, quercetin, and caffeic acid, as well as phenolic acids, in a test-tube investigation. If you'd like to get more of these antioxidants in your diet, dandelion tea is a great addition.

5. Milk: Loved by many, this beverage serves as a great source of antioxidants that fight disease in addition to increasing energy levels. Coffee is one of the main sources of antioxidants in the typical person's diet because some studies indicate that it contains even more effective antioxidant qualities than fruits and vegetables. Numerous antioxidants, including quercetin, catechin, caffeic acid, and rutin, are found in coffee.

A systematic analysis comprising 218 pieces of research found that consuming 3. 4–6 cups (720–960 mL) of coffee per day may reduce the incidence of liver issues, heart disease, and several cancers.

6. Pomegranate juice: Pomegranate is another product high in antioxidants. Based on certain study investigations, this fruit may have a higher antioxidant capacity than red wine and green tea. Pomegranate juice has also been shown in numerous trials to reduce blood pressure, reduce inflammation, and guard against the artery-clogging accumulation of fatty plaque.

Additionally, potassium, which is necessary for maintaining fluid balance, blood pressure, and muscular contractions, is abundant in pomegranates.

7. Beet Juice: Rich in phenolic compounds and essential antioxidants, beets have betalains, which are plant pigments that give them their vivid color. Beets provide numerous health benefits due to their antioxidant qualities, including lowering inflammation, strengthening the heart, and slowing the formation of malignant cells.

8. Acai Juice: Packed with powerful antioxidants including isoorientin, vanillic acid, and orientin, acai berries are a type of tropical berry. These days, you can find them in almost any health food store, but not too long ago, they were exclusively common in Central and South America.

For good reason, acai berries are frequently referred to as a "superfood. " In one study, for example, a small group of athletes found that, after just 1. 5 months, consuming a glass of juice infused with acai berries daily dramatically boosted blood antioxidant levels, decreased cholesterol, and helped repair muscle damage from exercise.

Acai juice may also lessen oxidative stress, enhance brain function, and stop bone loss, according to studies. To show this beyond a reasonable doubt, more research is necessary.

9. Juice (green): A variety of green vegetables, including kale, cucumber, parsley, and dill, are used to make green juice. Numerous vital antioxidants and micronutrients that are included in each of these substances have a substantial positive impact on health.

Cucumbers, for instance, have a high water content that aids in efficient digestion and helps you stay hydrated. They may also shield the body from the negative effects of diabetes. High concentrations of vitamin K and other antioxidants, such as quercetin and kaempferol, can be found in parsley. Numerous studies have examined the nutritional qualities of dill, and it has been demonstrated that using this substance can help manage heart disease and diabetes.

One easy method to boost your daily intake of antioxidants and give your body the nutrition it needs is to include a glass of green juice in your diet.

10. The green smoothie: Another delicious beverage that's loaded with antioxidants is a green smoothie. Typically, to balance out the flavor, sweet fruits and berries like bananas, strawberries, apples, or kiwis are blended with spinach, beet greens, alfalfa, and watercress.

11. Lemon Juice: Well-known for having a high vitamin C content, lemon juice is a great source of antioxidants. It has been demonstrated that vitamin C lowers the risk of stroke and heart disease. Lemons are also a good source of polyphenols, which are strong antioxidants that support healthy skin, aid in weight loss, and fight aging.

12. Water with cocoa: Micronutrients like manganese, potassium, and vitamin C are all abundant in coconut water. It has a significant antioxidant content as well. Animal studies have found that coconut water may help preserve liver health and lower blood sugar and oxidative stress, even if there hasn't been enough research done on humans. Try to find fresh coconut water while shopping, as opposed to canned and processed varieties, which have lower antioxidant counts.

How Can I Consume Sufficient Antioxidants Each Day?

You undoubtedly want to know how much of these antioxidant-rich beverages you need to drink in order to meet your daily dietary requirements. The following advice will assist you in ensuring that you consume a sufficient quantity of antioxidants each day.

Make as many dishes and ingredients as you can by hand rather than relying on store-bought items. In this manner, you will be in charge of what you eat. Consume healthy, complete foods and make an effort to increase your intake of fruits and vegetables. Select lean protein sources; Steer clear of harmful cooking techniques like deep-frying and microwaveing, as these methods dramatically reduce the nutritional content of food by heating at high temperatures and using large amounts of toxic oils. Arrange your food.

A FAQ
Do antioxidant drinks have any benefits?

Antioxidants can help prevent oxidative stress and a number of diseases, including diabetes, cancer, heart disease, arthritis, and stroke, if they are ingested from organic sources.

- What benefits do antioxidants offer the body? Antioxidants are substances that shield your body from free radical damage and stop cell deterioration, which can lead to cancer, heart disease, and other illnesses.

- Do antioxidants support the body's defenses?Antioxidants do have immune-boosting properties. Antioxidants have been shown in recent research to greatly enhance several immune responses. For instance, vitamin supplements containing E, C, and A aid in activating cells that protect the elderly from tumors.

- Is there an antioxidant in lemon juice?Yes, one of the greatest ways to get vitamin C, a powerful antioxidant, is to eat lemons and drink lemon juice.

- Are antioxidants truly effective?Antioxidants are indeed necessary for all living things. They both stop and postpone cell damage. It has been demonstrated that eating a diet high in fruits and vegetables, which are the primary sources of antioxidants, improves overall health and quality of life.

CHAPTER 5: Digestive Health Juices.

It goes without saying that juice for digestion can be a very effective treatment for troubled stomachs. This recipe for healthy gut juice, which includes beets, apples, celery, ginger, and apple vinegar, is not only delicious but also helps to soothe upset stomachs.

Fruit juices are well known for being an excellent indigestion remedy. When you have an upset stomach, juice might help soothe it and improve digestion.
Our digestive tracts need to be rested when we have stomach problems. It just means that we should not

be giving it as much labor. Thus, a juice diet is an excellent means of supporting overall health and helping with digestive issues.

These are some incredible natural juices that you may consume to help your digestive system function better.

1. Orange Smoothie with Aloe Vera and Spinach:
Citrus fruits contain citric acid. This is essential for lowering the possibility of a gastrointestinal upset. Oranges are also a great source of soluble fiber, which coats your intestinal walls like a gel. Your body can more effectively absorb the nutrients as a result. Smoodies is a source of 100% natural orange juice.
You can be sure you're getting all the nutrients your body needs by adding spinach juice to the beverage. Enzymes and other nutrients included in aloe vera juice can aid in eliminating toxins and cleansing your digestive tract.

2. Smoothie with pineapple and cucumber:
Bromelain, an enzyme found in pineapple juice or smoothies, ensures that any gastrointestinal discomfort is alleviated. Cucumber guarantees that

the juice cools down your digestive tract. This is very useful during the summer.

3. Smoothie with apples, cucumbers, and lettuce: Fennel seeds mixed with apple juice can help reduce any irritation in your digestive tract. Additionally, it treats intestinal burns. In addition, cucumbers are rich in enzymes that aid in the elimination of toxins from the body. You can be certain that the smoothie won't cause acid reflux if it contains lettuce. Similar gastrointestinal issues, like heartburn, can also be prevented.

4. Smoothie with green apples and cucumbers: Another fantastic fruit that can aid with digestive problems is the green apple. The juice may help facilitate regular bowel motions. This lowers the chance of colon cancer as well. The cucumber in the smoothie will help cool down your digestive tract.

5. Lime juice: Having a daily glass of lemonade in the morning will benefit your digestive system. It gets rid of any poisons that are in your body. You can even prevent any liver issues with this method. Lemonade can aid with weight control in addition to promoting good digestion. Lemonade can aid with digestive problems, and tulsi increases immunity.

6. Granola Juice: Another beverage that may be good for your digestive tract is pomegranate juice. It lessens intestinal irritation. Your ability to digest food improves significantly. Those who have ulcers or inflammatory bowel disease can greatly benefit from pomegranate juice.
Smoodies is a source for genuine pomegranate juice. It is also a great source of vitamin C and can help lower blood pressure.

7. Mango Juice: Green Mangos are a great source of essential minerals, including vitamins A and C. By consuming this drink, you can prevent dehydration. More significantly, raw mango juice is beneficial for a number of stomach ailments. Green mango juice can assist with digestive disorders such as diarrhea, bloating, and constipation.
Smoodies are available with green mango juice. Your digestive tract may be stimulated by the mango juice. Digestion-related heat is dissipated with the help of this secretion of digestive enzymes.

Smoodies offers a large selection of juices that can support numerous health advantages and general well-being. All fruit is used to make the juices; no extra sugar or preservatives are used.

A toxin is an organic poison that occurs naturally and is created by the metabolic processes of living things. The two main categories of toxins are internal and external. Internal toxins include urea, lactic acid, and waste products naturally created by gut bacteria during metabolism. Toxins from the outside might enter our bodies through the skin, food, drink, or respiration. Your body can absorb toxins through your skin, food, drink, or respiration. Toxins are also produced by your body's metabolic activities. Your body breaks down and gets rid of these toxins when you exercise.

CHAPTER 6: Energy and Nutrient-Dense Juices.

All foods provide energy, but there are wide differences in the ways they impact the body. While grains, legumes, and complete foods offer more sustained energy that will keep the body functioning longer, sugars and refined carbohydrates only offer a momentary boost.

The list we provide here is concentrated on foods and beverages that offer more consistent energy levels throughout the day.

FRUITS

The ensuing fruits could provide an energy boost.

1. Bananas: Potassium is abundant in bananas. Perhaps the greatest quick snack for long-lasting energy is a banana. Bananas are a fantastic natural source of sugar, but they also contain a lot of fiber, which slows down the sugar's digestion. Beneficial nutrients included in bananas give the body a boost of energy.

Just like a carbohydrate drink, eating a banana before a long bike ride improves performance and endurance. Bananas can still supply you with energy, even if most individuals don't ride their bikes every day.

2. Avocados: Rich in nutrients and health benefits, avocados are a fruit that has it all.
According to research published in Critical Reviews in Food Science and Nutrition, they provide fiber, protein, and minerals that could help maintain energy levels all day.

Additionally, they include healthy fats that may boost energy levels and improve the body's availability of fat-soluble nutrients.

3. Goji Berries: According to a review in Drug Design, Development, and Therapy notes, goji berries are tiny, reddish berries with a wealth of nutrients and significant anti-aging and antioxidant qualities. The body may benefit from the particular antioxidants in several ways, including increased energy.

Many people add some dried goji berries to a water bottle to sip during the day, and they also make a terrific addition to trail mixes.

4. Apples: Another easy snack that could provide the body with sustained energy is an apple. According to research published in the journal Horticulture Research, apples are a good source of flavonoids, which are antioxidants that can help prevent inflammation and oxidative stress in the body.

5. Strawberries are a good source of minerals, vitamin C, and folates, according to a study published in the Journal of Agricultural and Food Chemistry.

They also include phenols, which are vital antioxidants that might aid in the body's cellular synthesis of energy.
Strawberries can be added to a lot of different recipes, and they can also be a simple diet snack.

6. Oranges: The taste of oranges is attributed to the antioxidant vitamin C, which is why most people like them. Vitamin C may aid in preventing fatigue and lowering oxidative stress in the body.

Young adult male students who have greater amounts of vitamin C may also be happier and less prone to experience bewilderment, rage, or despair, according to a study published in the journal Antioxidants.

7. Dark berries: When the body is yearning for something sweet, berries like blueberries, raspberries, and blackberries may be an excellent food to enhance energy.

Compared to lighter-colored berries, dark berries typically contain more natural antioxidants, which may lessen weariness and inflammation in the body.

They satisfy a sweet taste need while also typically containing less sugar than tastier fruits.

ANIMATED GOODS:

The following animal-based foods could provide you with more energy:

8. Fatty fish: Omega-3 fatty acids, which are found in salmon, may enhance cognitive performance and lessen tiredness. In general, fish is a great, low-calorie source of B vitamins and protein that can help the body maintain energy levels throughout the day.

Omega-3 fatty acids are typically found in larger concentrations in fatty cold-water fish like tuna, sardines, and salmon.
Omega-3 fatty acids may lessen inflammation in the body and enhance brain function, both of which may contribute to exhaustion in certain individuals.

9. Beef liver: High in vitamin B-12, which keeps the body feeling energized, beef liver may be one of the greatest meat sources.

Although vitamin B-12 is present in various meat cuts, beef liver has a higher concentration than other meat cuts.

The United States Department of Agriculture (USDA) estimates that the vitamin B-12 content of a 3-ounce portion of beef flank steak is around 1. 5 micrograms (mcg).
The USDA states that the same cut of beef liver has 60 mcg of vitamin B-12 (trusted source).

10. Yogurt: Another potential energy source is yogurt. Natural yogurt is high in protein, lipids, and simple carbs, all of which give the body energy, as the USDA indicates.
Yogurt is a fantastic substitute for meals from vending machines because it's convenient to eat on the go.

11. Eggs: Rich in protein and other minerals, eggs give the body energy that lasts. According to the USDA, a big hard-boiled egg has roughly 6 grams (g) of protein and 5 grams of fat (trusted source), along with vitamins and minerals that help the body stay fuller and more energetic for longer than other snacks.

VEGETABLES

The following types of vegetables are high in energy:

12. Sweet potatoes and yams. Sweet potatoes and yams are good sources of carbs, which provide you with energy. However, sweet potatoes also include a lot of fiber, which could help slow down how quickly the body absorbs these carbohydrates. They can therefore be an excellent choice if you want energy that lasts all day.

13. Beets: According to research published in the journal Food Science and Biotechnology, beets may be a fantastic source of minerals and antioxidants for the body, which can enhance blood flow and vitality. Beets can be eaten raw, cooked, or in the form of a bottle of beetroot juice.

14. Dark green vegetables. Leafy greens that are dark in color, like spinach, kale, and collard greens, are rich in nutrients and antioxidants, and they also contain filling proteins.

Some people may find it difficult to digest greens raw, so cooking them with a little vinegar or lemon juice can help break them down.

15. Dark chocolate: Eating dark chocolate could be a simple method of boosting energy. Compared to milk chocolate, rich, dark chocolate typically contains substantially less sugar. Reduced sugar content results in less immediate energy, but increased cocoa content yields more cocoa benefits, including protective antioxidants like flavonoids.

According to a study published in the Archives of the Turkish Society of Cardiology journal, eating dark chocolate may improve cardiovascular health by increasing blood flow throughout the body. Fresh oxygen carried by this blood may also help an individual feel more awake and aware.

GRAINS

The ensuing grains could provide you with more energy.

16. Oatmeal: A bowl of whole-grain oatmeal could be a fantastic source of energy for the body.

Because of their high fiber content, oats may help the body feel fuller for longer than other breakfast options.

Whole-grain oats are also a source of important minerals, vitamins, and phenolic compounds, all of which may help energize the body, according to a study published in The Journal of Nutrition.

17. Popcorn: A good source of carbs is popcorn. To aid in slowing down digestion, it also contains fiber. Compared to other carbohydrates, popcorn might help someone feel fuller for longer.

As a study in the Nutrition Journal notes, people who ate popcorn rather than potato chips felt fuller from the snack. This may be helpful for dieters, as popcorn usually contains fewer calories than potato chips.

18. Quinoa: Quinoa is a seed, yet most people treat it as a grain. Quinoa is high in protein, carbs, and fiber. The combination of amino acids and slow-release carbs may make for lasting energy rather than a fast burst of glucose from other grains.

19. Brown rice: One of the benefits of brown rice may be that it preserves much of the fiber from the husk. The husk is not there in white rice, which may cause the body to absorb the carbohydrate content quicker.

This may lead to a spike and then a drop in energy levels. By possessing the husk, brown rice may help slow the digestion of these carbohydrates, therefore releasing energy more slowly.

BEANS AND LEGUMES

The following beans and legumes may aid with energy:

20. Soybeans: Whether roasted soybeans or young edamame beans in the pod, soybeans contain protein with a wide array of amino acids, as well as magnesium and potassium, according to the USDA.

21. Lentils: Lentils are a wonderful source of protein and fiber. Lentils are a relatively cheap kind of protein and fiber, which may make them an excellent alternative for folks on a budget.

The USDA reports that 1 cup of lentils has roughly 18 g of protein, 40 g of carbs, 15 g of fiber, and less than 4 g of sugar.

The fiber may aid in controlling the digestion of the carbs, keeping the body full, and providing a source of prolonged energy.

22. Nuts: Many nuts contain a blend of protein, lipids, and some carbohydrates to offer energy throughout the day. A typical nut's abundance of vitamins and minerals includes calcium, phosphorus, and magnesium.
Nuts often contain large amounts of important fatty acids.

According to research published in the Journal of Parenteral and Enteral Nutrition, these fats have the potential to lessen inflammation, which in turn may lessen weariness.
Additionally, nuts are heavy in calories; therefore, consumers should use caution while consuming them.

23. Peanut butter: Packed with fiber, protein, and lipids, peanut butter can help you feel fuller for longer after eating it. This could reduce the need for frequent eating, which can wear someone out because their body is always breaking down food.

24. Seeds: A lot of seeds, including chia, flax, and pumpkin seeds, are high in fatty acids and fiber, which may provide you with extra energy. In addition to being convenient to carry, seeds are a fantastic component of a trail mix.

DRINKS

The energy-boosting beverages listed below include:

25. Water: Of all the ingredients on this list, water is the most essential for energy. Every cell in the body needs water to function properly.
Although most people consider dehydration to be an extreme situation, if someone goes without water for the entire morning, their body may get somewhat dehydrated.

Keeping a water bottle with you and drinking from it throughout the day might help you stay well hydrated and sustain your energy.

26. Coffee: It's common knowledge that coffee increases energy. Caffeine, which is included in coffee, alerts the body and mind and may increase productivity.
Additionally, coffee has antioxidants called polyphenols that may help the body function better by lowering oxidative stress in the cells.

But since coffee is a stimulant, people ought to drink it sparingly. Loss of energy may result from consuming too much coffee as the body adjusts to the caffeine.

27. Green tea: Although it still has trace quantities of caffeine, green tea also contains chemicals that may help lower inflammation and oxidative stress in the body. As a result, it can be easier to go from a more alert and energized state to coffee.

28. Yerba maté: This South American beverage is indigenous. The body experiences comparable stimulating effects from drinking the herb or tea as it does from coffee or tea.

Amino acids, antioxidants, and other active nutrients are abundant in yerba maté. Those who use yerba maté claim that it offers a far more gradual source of energy than the burst of energy found in coffee.

According to a study published in the journal Nutrients, yerba maté may also make people feel happier and more satisfied—even after working out—which could be advantageous for those trying to reduce weight without sacrificing energy.

Avoidable Foods:

Though numerous foods provide you with energy, the ones listed above concentrate on long-lasting energy.

Items to attempt to stay away from include:
- Fried or quick food items.
- Extra sugars.
- Candy bars and packed snacks. Cakes and cupcakes are examples of baked treats.

Consuming a diversified, balanced diet is the purpose behind finding foods that promote energy, even though this list is not all-inclusive. Finding a

balance between vitamins, fiber, fats, and proteins is vital for energy production.
People should make an effort to pick a diversified diet that includes a wide variety of nourishing meals that provide the body with sustained energy.

CHAPTER 7: Hydration And Detoxification.

We come into contact with artificial chemicals, poisonous materials, contaminated water, processed foods, pollution in the environment, and other things that make us susceptible to disease on a daily basis. Thankfully, the body has self-regulating systems in place to get rid of pollutants and bring things back into harmony. These self-regulatory systems can occasionally get overloaded with substances, infections, and environmental toxins, which impairs their ability to operate and causes disease or a low mood.

However, you may help your body's natural detoxification process and restore its equilibrium by making a few small changes.
It is inevitable to be exposed to harmful toxins, even in our own bodies. Despite the fact that our bodies have an effective metabolic detoxification mechanism that neutralizes and gets rid of dangerous poisons, we are exposed to contaminants in food, water, and the air. We are frequently exposed to a variety of poisons, including pesticides, heavy metals, volatile chemical compounds, and persistent organic pollutants.

These contaminants have the potential to accumulate over time and weaken the detoxification system, which can result in disease and other health issues. Even if it's not feasible to completely avoid environmental pollutants, we can try our best to provide our detoxification system with the resources it needs to perform at its best.

The System of Natural Detoxification.

Numerous organs in the human body cooperate to aid in detoxification.

These consist of:

1. The Liver: The liver is located under the rib cage and on the upper right side of the abdomen. The liver is essential to life and performs a variety of vital functions in the body. It is in charge of more than 500 recognized functions, **such as:**

a. Bile production: The liver produces bile, a green or yellow fluid, in order to break down dietary fat.
Although the liver produces it, the gallbladder stores and concentrates it. It is also in charge of transporting waste products from the liver and intestines for elimination.

b. Glucose's transformation into glycogen: The body uses the liver to transform the glucose in food into glycogen, which is then stored and has the potential to be turned back into glucose when needed. control of amino acid synthesis to produce protein Iron store processing of hemoglobin. Control of coagulation factorsproduction of defense mechanism.

Removal of bilirubin An orange-yellow material called bilirubin is created when red blood cells break down. It is eliminated from the body after passing through the liver.

c. Remove poisons: The liver is in charge of removing chemicals, medications, and poisons from the blood. Ammonia's transformation into urea One byproduct of protein metabolism is ammonia. The liver transforms ammonia into urea, which is subsequently eliminated by the urinary tract.

2. The kidneys: They are two bean-shaped organs situated beneath the rib cage on either side. An essential component of the body's natural detoxification process are the kidneys. Every minute, they filter about a half cup of blood, eliminating waste and surplus water to produce urine. The entire urinary system is formed when the pee travels via the ureters and into the bladder.

In addition, the kidneys eliminate acid generated by biological processes and preserve the right amounts of water, salt, and minerals in the body—many of which are essential for healthy tissues, muscle, and nerve function. The hormones that the kidneys generate both control blood pressure and the production of red blood cells.

The glomerulus and tubule found in nephrons, which make up the kidney's filtration system, are structures. The tubule adds nutrients to the blood and eliminates waste, while the glomerulus filters the blood. Only approximately one or two quarters of the 150 quarts of blood that the kidneys filter each day end up as urine. The blood receives the majority of its water and nutrition back.

3. The Intestines: The intestines are an essential component of the immune system and digestive system. The small and big intestines are two distinct organ systems that are included in the intestines. The ileum, jejunum, and duodenum comprise the small intestine. The rectum, colon, cecum, and appendix make up the large intestine. The intestines work in tandem to break down food into nutrients like proteins, lipids, carbs, minerals, and vitamins. These nutrients are essential for growth and energy production since they break down proteins into amino acids, which power brain and muscle development.

Additionally, the intestines support the immune system. To prevent harmful bacteria, parasites, and other substances from entering the bloodstream, the small intestine's lymph nodes fight these intruders.

4. The Skin: The largest organ in the body and the body's first line of defense against toxins is the skin. The skin works as a barrier to keep many poisons from entering our systems, even though it absorbs many toxins, including those found in clothing, cosmetics, and contaminated air.
The kidneys receive support from the skin to enable optimal renal function. Crystal waste products are eliminated, along with excess refined sugar and acidic foods. Protein-rich diets include dairy and meat.

5. The lymphatic system: Is made up of lymph nodes, lymph ducts, and thin-walled lymphatic veins. It is a component of the immune system. The lymph fluid that the veins carry throughout the body gives tissues the essential nutrition they need to function.

Additionally, lymph passes through lymph nodes, which allow waste materials from cells to be filtered and removed from the venous flow. White blood cells, or lymphocytes, are another type of immune cell produced by lymph nodes and are used to fight off bacteria, viruses, and other foreign invaders. Veins receive the contents of the ducts into which lymph vessels empty.

Helping Your System of Detoxification.

The detoxification system functions efficiently on its own in healthy bodies to preserve harmony and balance. But when the organs are overworked, they become exhausted and require a bit more assistance. By providing your body with the support it needs, **you can naturally detox in the following ways:**

1. A nutritious diet is essential to maintaining the health of your systems and organs.
2. Processed foods include refined sugars, artificial coloring, additives, and preservatives, among other chemicals and contaminants that interfere with your body's natural detoxification process.
3. Add each and every one of the following foods to your diet to help your body's detoxification process:
4. consuming five to nine portions of fresh produce every day. Consuming whole grains, nuts, and seeds to get fiberselecting berries, artichokes, garlic, leeks, and cruciferous veggies like broccoli, spinach, and
5. Brussels sprouts.
6. Consuming grass-fed animals that are high in lean protein.
7. Consuming fermented foods for gut health, such as kefir, sauerkraut, kimchi, and yogurt.

Hydration is necessary for all of the body's detoxification systems and organs, as you can see, as they depend on blood or fluid flow to be flushed out. The human body needs a sufficient volume of fluid to operate at its best overall, especially when it comes to kidney function and blood volume circulation. In fact, some research indicates that chronic dehydration—even in moderate forms—may cause irreversible kidney damage.

Dehydration makes it harder for the kidneys to filter waste, which increases the risk of kidney stones and urinary tract infections.
We lose water every day by breathing, perspiring, peeing, and even sweating. We get dehydrated if that water isn't replaced. Along with the fluids, we're also losing electrolytes, including magnesium, chloride, potassium, and sodium.

Although there isn't a universally accepted amount of water that is considered optimal, you can keep an eye on your own hydration levels by being aware of how you feel.

- Urine testing is the most reliable method of determining your level of hydration.
- Urine that is dark and concentrated suggests dehydration.
- You are well hydrated if your urine is pale. You need to replenish your electrolytes if your pee is clear or almost clear.

Our meals provide us with various electrolytes, primarily sodium, but unbalanced or bad diets can cause deficits in specific electrolytes, including magnesium. You can take an electrolyte supplement to restore your electrolyte balance and provide your body with the minerals it needs if you're worried about it.

Buoy can assist you in bolstering your body's detoxifying system. You can add the portable and squeezable electrolyte supplement to your preferred beverage to receive a quick energy boost while on the road. (any beverage!!). Squeeze your buoy for immediate sustenance, whether you're working out hard and sweating or searching for a method to add critical nutrients to your diet.

CHAPTER 8: Smoothies And Blended Recipes Options.

For anyone searching for a quick and wholesome lunch or snack, healthy smoothie recipes are an essential carry-along. They're loaded with fruits and vegetables, really simple to create, and done in a matter of seconds. Still, not every smoothie will assist you in achieving your dietary objectives. In actuality, a lot of smoothies from the shop have a lot of added sugar.

These delicious smoothie recipes will go well with your morning meals, whether you want a deep chocolate recipe or the traditional strawberry one. And to ensure that you always have the ideal consistency when preparing these delicious dishes, utilize one of the greatest smoothie blenders available.

Smoothies with an appropriate ratio of nutrients and ingredients, such as protein, carbohydrates, and healthy fats, can serve as a nutritious breakfast option.

Adding extra fiber from veggies, flax, hemp, or chia seeds, as well as a source of healthy fat like almonds or avocado, can also help supply important vitamins, minerals, and antioxidants, the expert says.

Is drinking a smoothie every day healthy?
If you want to start preparing smoothies at home with your own blender, you've already taken the first step toward controlling what goes into your drink and saving money. Consuming a smoothie on a daily basis is perfectly fine as long as the nutritional composition is balanced.
With probiotic-rich yogurt, creamy milk, protein, and other nutrient-dense ingredients, these tasty and nutritious smoothies make eating well easier.

A word of caution: You can omit the fruit juice or honey listed in any of these recipes if you're trying to reduce your intake of added sugar.

1. Bowl of Blueberry:

SmoothieWho says smoothies aren't meant to be consumed? Blend almond butter, frozen blueberries, almond milk, and vanilla until the mixture is incredibly smooth and delicious. For the breakfast bowl of your dreams, garnish after dividing into two bowls with hemp seeds, vanilla granola, fresh blueberries, and other toppings.

2. Shake with Berries, Chia, and Mint:
This ruby smoothie, which is loaded with strawberries, raspberries, and beets, has our favorite color—red. You'll get a ton of fiber that is good for your gut, along with a pleasant sip from the unexpected mint inclusion.

3. Coconut Pineapple Green Smoothie:
Baby spinach adds nutrients and tropical tastes from pineapple, coconut, banana, and lime. This nutrient-dense cup is perfect for any time of day and tastes like an island vacation.

4. Smoothies for Less Stress:
The gut-boosting properties of tart kefir, when paired with hemp seeds, raspberries, and peaches, may help reduce stress. If hemp seeds are unavailable, you may still get a similar magnesium

boost by adding a spoonful of almond butter. Magnesium is important for reducing stress.

5. Luscious Kale Smoothie:

This smoothie is found in Prevention's Smoothies & Juices section under Balanced Gut. Greek yogurt is an excellent source of probiotics and protein, which naturally improve intestinal health.

1 cup of roughly chopped kale, 1 1/2 cups of frozen pineapple chunks, 1/2 cup of plain Greek yogurt, 1/2 cup of unsweetened almond milk, and 1 teaspoon of honey should all be combined in a blender. Blend the mixture until it becomes foamy and smooth.

Nutrition: 8.5 g fat (3 g sat fat), 36 g sugars (6 g added sugars), 5 g fiber, 45 g carb, and 296 cal.

6. Pineapple-Citrus Smoothie Bowl:

This healthy smoothie bowl is a great way to mix things up. It has heart-healthy cashews, gut-healthy Greek yogurt, and vitamin C-rich citrus fruit. Blend together half a cup fat-free Greek yogurt, half a cup frozen pineapple chunks, a teaspoon vanilla essence, half a navel orange, and half a ruby grapefruit. After blending until smooth, divide the mixture into two bowls. Add extra orange and grapefruit on top, along with chopped cashews, chia seeds, and unsweetened coconut flakes.

Nutrition: 240 calories, 12 g protein, 31 g carbohydrates, 5 g fiber, 19 g sugars (with 0 g added sugars), and 8 g fat (with 4 g sat fat).

6. Blueberry Peach Smoothie:

With its sweet balance of peaches and blueberries, this combination will make you feel like it's summer even in the dead of winter. Plus, the nutrient-dense kale will provide you with your recommended daily intake of greens. The ideal finishing touch is a dash of cinnamon.

In a blender, add 1 cup chilled almond or vanilla soy milk, 4 slices of fresh or frozen peaches (approximately 1/2 cup), 1/4 cup blueberries, a handful of kale, and 1/4 tsp. cinnamon powder. Mix until homogeneous.

Nutrition: 170 calories, 8.5 g protein, 26 g carbohydrates, 4 g fiber, 17 g sugars, and 4 g fat.

8. Blueberry-banana-soy Smoothie:

This nutritious smoothie has plenty of flavor from succulent blueberries, enhanced by the addition of potassium-rich bananas and vanilla for sweetness. Just mix 1/2 cup frozen blueberries, 1/2 frozen banana, and 1 teaspoon pure vanilla extract with 1 1/4 cups light soy milk. Blend until smooth, about 20 to 30 seconds. If you would like a thinner mixture, you can add up to 1/4 cup extra milk.

Protein: 3 g, carbohydrates: 25 g, fiber: 2 g, sugars: 11 g, fat: 5 g.

9. Smoothie with Peaches and Cream Oatmeal:
Too busy to have a leisurely meal? Try this quick and easy, high-probiotic version of oatmeal in the morning. Prebiotic fiber, which is included in whole-grain oats, helps to maintain intestinal health.

Blend 1/2 cup whole milk, 1/2 cup Greek yogurt, 1/2 cup rolled oats, 1 cup frozen peaches, 1/2 frozen banana, and 1/2 cup ice until smooth. This recipe from Prevention's Smoothies & Juices prepares two smoothies.

Nutrition: 283 calories, 13 g protein, 53.5 g carbohydrates, 2 g fiber, 48 g sugars, and 3.5 g fat (2 g saturated fat).

10. Smoothie with Pineapple: PassionYour need for an ice cream cone will be satisfied by this lusciously thick smoothie recipe. Furthermore, pineapple has an enzyme called bromelain that aids in the breakdown of proteins and may lessen bloating.
Mix one cup of pineapple chunks, six ice cubes, and one cup of light or low-fat vanilla yogurt. In a blender, combine all the ingredients and pulse until smooth, adding more as needed.

Nutrition: 283 calories, 13 g protein, 53.5 g carbohydrates, 2 g fiber, 48 g sugars, and 3.5 g fat (2 g saturated fat).

11. Honey and Milk Smoothie: This blended juice is a great way to use up the celery you have in your vegetable drawer. It tastes great served as a snack with grapes, cucumber, and almond milk.
One medium Kirby cucumber (peeled and sliced), one cup seedless green grapes, two medium stalks of celery (peeled and sliced), and one tablespoon honey

should all be combined in a blender. Process until smooth; this makes two servings.

Nutrition: 2 g protein, 26 g carbohydrates, 2 g fiber, 21 g sugars (9 g added sugars), 2 g fat (0 g saturated fat).

12. Smoothy Skin Drink:
This beverage is excellent for your complexion and comes from Prevention's Smoothies and Juices! Carrots and apricots are high in beta-carotene, an antioxidant that the body uses to make vitamin A. The vitamin may be able to prevent pollution and UV damage, as well as premature aging of the skin. Mix 1/2 cup ice cubes, 1/2 cup Greek yogurt with whole milk, 1/4 cup shredded carrot, 1 tsp honey, 1/2 tsp cinnamon, 2 chopped dried apricots, and 1 chopped fresh apricot (pitted and finely diced) in a blender. Mix until homogeneous.

Nutrition: 130 calories, 8 g protein, 21 g carbohydrates, 3 g fiber, 17 g sugars (6 g added sugars), 3.5 g fat (2 g sat fat),

13: Green, Lean, and Mean Machine:

This smoothie is perfect if you're seeking a post-workout recovery beverage. Protein powder aids in restoring burned energy; potassium and vitamin C are provided by sweet bananas and kiwis; and hydration is assisted by coconut water.

Add one medium banana, one peeled and chopped kiwi, one cup unsweetened almond milk, one cup spinach, one scoop vanilla whey protein powder, and half a cup coconut water to a blender. Blend until smooth and creamy.
304 calories, 22 g protein, 47 g carbohydrates, 7 g fiber, and 5 g fat.

14. Fruit, Banana, and Oat Smoothie:
Smoothies gain body from oats, and their resistant starch content keeps you feeling full for longer. An additional benefit of resistant starch Compared to other fibers, it produces less gas.
Blend together 2 cups frozen strawberries, 1 cup low-fat vanilla yogurt, 1 sliced banana, 1/2 cup rolled oats, 1/2 cup orange juice, and 1 tablespoon honey in a blender. Process until smooth; this makes 4 servings.

Nutrition: 171 calories, 5 g protein, 36 g carbohydrates, 3.5 g fiber, 23 g sugars (4.5 g added sugars), 2 g fat (1 g sat fat).

15. Dreamy Caribbean Smoothie:

If you frequently experience nausea before important occasions, consider consuming this smoothie from Prevention's Smoothies & Juices. It has bananas, which are high in the calming mineral magnesium, and the bacteria in the yogurt can help reduce anxiety.

To make a smooth smoothie, blend together 1/2 cup pineapple chunks, 1/4 cup Greek yogurt, 1/4 cup chilled unsweetened coconut milk, 1/4 cup orange juice, 1/4 large banana, and a few ice cubes. If you want to reduce anxiety as much as possible, try drinking it two hours before you need to relax.

Nutrition: 21 g sugars (1.5 g added sugars), 3 g fat (2 g sat fat), 6 g pro, 29 g carb, 2 g fiber, and 156 calories.

16. Ginger Green Smoothie:

The vibrant green hue of this smoothie is a result of the combination of baby spinach and Granny Smith apples. Hemp seeds offer a healthy fat- and plant-based protein boost.

Add 1 diced Granny Smith apple, 2 cups packed baby spinach, 3/4 cup coconut water, 1/4 cup lemon juice, and 2 tablespoons of coconut oil. three tablespoons of hemp seeds. one tablespoon of finely chopped ginger. one-half cup ice cubes, raw honey. Mix until homogeneous. This dish serves two.

Nutrition: 17 g sugars, 4 g fiber, 27 g carbs, and 4 g fat (1 g saturated fat) make up the nutrition.

17. Banana and Cranberry Smoothie:
This filling, high-fiber treat's star is the autumn berry. Almond milk cuts calories, bananas lend body and sweetness, and maple syrup adds a touch of seasonal sweetness.
Put one cup of frozen cranberries, one cup of unsweetened almond milk, one banana, and one tablespoon into a blender. frozen cubes and ½ cup maple syrup. Blend until smooth and foamy.

Nutrition: 1 g pro, 27 g carb, 4 g fiber, 15.5 g sugars (of which 6 g are added), and 1.5 g fat (of which 0 g is saturated fat).

18. A Crisp Apple Juice:

This smoothie, made with sweet apple cider, Greek yogurt, oats, almonds, and comforting spices, is a great way to enjoy the flavors of fall. Moreover, it contains a lot of protein and beta-glucan, a fiber type that increases stamina.

Nutrition: 364 calories, 14 g protein, 49 g carbohydrates, 4 g fiber, 32 g sugars, and 12.5 g fat (2 g sat fat).

19. Smoothie With Green Tea:

blueberries, and bananasJust warm up 3 tablespoons of green tea to make this antioxidant-rich smoothie. Heat a bowl of water in the microwave until it's piping hot. After that, add 1 green tea bag and give it 3 minutes to brew. Take out the tea bag and add two teaspoons of honey until it dissolves. In a blender, combine 1 1/2 cups frozen blueberries, 1/2 medium banana, and 3/4 cup light vanilla soy milk with calcium fortification. When all the ingredients are blended, add the tea.

Nutrition: 38.5 g sugars, 2.5 g fat (g sat fat), 63 g carbs, 8 g fiber, and 269 calories.

20. Shake Mocha Protein:
This jittery breakfast has a milkshake-like flavor.
The key component is almonds. These nuts are rich
in protein and heart-healthy omega-3 fatty acids,
which have been shown to reduce inflammation and
safeguard the heart. This is the ideal morning shake,
thanks to the addition of black coffee.

Place one large frozen banana (cut into bits), one
cup of ice cubes, one-half cup of premade and
cooled black coffee, one-fourth cup of walnuts, and
one heaping tablespoon into a blender. Add 6
tablespoons of unsweetened cocoa powder.
powdered chocolate protein. Mix until
homogeneous. There are two servings per recipe.
264 calories, 24 g protein, 22 g carbohydrates, 4 g
fiber, and 11 g fat

21. Supercharged Pumpkin Shake:
Greek yogurt is added to the pure pumpkin in this
smoothie to create a creamy, protein-rich base.
Seasonal sweetness is added with pumpkin pie spice
and maple syrup.
Put 1/2 cup canned pure pumpkin (frozen in an ice
cube tray) and 7 ounces of water into a blender. 1/4

avocado, 1/2 cup water, 2% Greek yogurt, and 2 Tbsp. 1 tablespoon ground flaxseed with 1/2 tsp. of maple syrup. spice for pumpkin pie. Until creamy, blend.

Nutrition: 361 calories, 26 g protein, 38 g carbohydrates, 11 g fiber, 26 g sugars, and 14 g fat (sat fat).

22. Kiwi-Strawberry Smoothie:

Using organic kiwis, which have higher levels of heart-healthy polyphenols and vitamin C, makes this tasty, low-calorie smoothie recipe even healthier. Blend together 1 ripe banana, 1 kiwi, 5 frozen strawberries, 1 1/4 cups cold apple juice, and 1 1/2 teaspoons honey in a blender. Blend until homogenous.

Nutrition: 16.5 g sugars, 0 g fat, 1.5 g fiber, 22 g carbs, 0.5 g protein.

23. Smoothie with Tropical Papaya Perfection:

This breakfast smoothie with coconut flavor is every bit as rich as a milkshake. You'll be transported to a tropical island with only one drink.

Dice one papaya and combine it with one cup fat-free plain yogurt, one-half cup fresh pineapple pieces, one-half cup crushed ice, and one teaspoon of honey. one teaspoon, and coconut extract. crush the flaxseed. Blend the mixture for approximately 30 seconds, or until it becomes frosty and smooth.

Nutrition: 299 calories, 8 g fiber, 64 g carbs, 13 g protein, 44 g sugars, and 1.5 g fat.

24. Almond and Banana Protein Smoothie:

After a strenuous workout, coconut water helps replenish electrolytes, while creamy almond butter provides healthy fats. A scoop of whey and Greek yogurt maintain a high protein content.
Add 3 tablespoons, 1/2 cup plain Greek yogurt, and 1/2 cup coconut water to a blender. almond butter, one tablespoon, and one scoop of whey protein powder. one frozen banana, one cup of ice, and hemp seeds. Blend until silky. This recipe yields two servings.

Nutrition: 15 g sugars, 17 g fat, 5 g fiber, 26 g carbs, and 329 calories.

25. Berry-Based Healthy Workout Drink:

With the help of this simple smoothie recipe, you may have the energy you need to finish your workout in no time. Consider adding a teaspoon of organic kale powder for an additional calcium boost. 1 1/2 cups cut strawberries, 1 cup blueberries, 1/2 cup raspberries, and 2 Tbsp are required. 1 teaspoon honey half a cup of ice cubes and fresh lemon juice. Mix until homogeneous.

162 calories, 2 grams of protein, 41.5 grams of carbohydrates, 6 grams of fiber, 32 grams of sugar, and 1 gram of fat

26th. Juicy Tutti-FruttiThis nutritious and reviving snack gets a citrus boost with a dash of orange juice. All you need is 1/2 cup of orange juice, 1/2 cup of plain yogurt, 1/2 cup of sliced ripe banana, 1/2 cup of canned crushed pineapple in juice, and 1/2 cup of mixed frozen berries. Process until smooth, about 2 minutes. This dish serves two. (If you want to reduce the amount of sugar, use fresh pineapple instead of canned or orange juice.)

Nutrition: 140 kcal, 3.5 g pro, 29 g carb, 2.5 g fiber, 16 g sugars, 2.5 g fat (1.5 g saturated fat).

26. Crazy Mango Smoothie:

Benefit from the anti-disease properties of ripe mangos by making this delectable smoothie recipe. First, put one large peeled and pitted mango, one ripe banana, one can of juice-packed pineapple pieces, and one cup of fat-free frozen vanilla yogurt in a blender. Mix until homogeneous. Next, add 4 cups of ice at a time until the mixture is completely pureed. The end product is a frozen, creamy beverage that's ideal for two people.

Nutrition: 0.5 g fat, 50 g sugars, 60 g carbs, 4 g fiber, and 251 calories.

27. Smoothie with Sweet Potato Puree:

This delicious smoothie is high in protein, fiber, and good fats. Along with its rich, nutty flavor and creamy texture, this breakfast food's vibrant yellow color (a result of the immune-boosting vitamin A) is sure to make your morning more cheerful.

Nutrition: 17 g protein, 68 g carbohydrates, 10 g fiber, 28 g sugars, and 13 g fat in 448 calories.

28. Gingerbread Smoothie to Go:

With nearly 30 g of protein per serving, this recipe is perfect if you're seeking a protein boost in the morning. In addition, it's a delightful treat that differs slightly from traditional smoothies made with fruits or vegetables. It tastes like a Christmas dessert in a cup since it's loaded with almond butter, frozen bananas, molasses, and spices like nutmeg, cinnamon, and ginger!

Nutrition: 440 calories, 27 g protein, 39 g carbohydrates, 5.5 g fiber, 30 g sugars, and 20 g fat.

29. Smoothie with Blackberry Nut Butter:

This easy recipe is perfect for a hectic morning or a quick lunch on-the-go because it only requires four ingredients and can be made in about five minutes. All you'll need are your favorite nut butter (almond or peanut butter works well), milk, honey, and blackberries. After that, combine and enjoy!

Nutrition: 53 g sugars, 10 g fat, 63 g carbs, 21 g protein, and 93 calories.

30. Smoothie with Kiwifruit and Silky Tofu:

This recipe's tofu creates a very satisfying, high-protein smoothie, and the kiwi gives each cup a zesty, invigorating taste. This is a tasty and nutritious alternative to most other smoothie recipes because it contains less sugar and fat.

Nutrition: 200 calories, 17 g protein, 31 g carbohydrates, 3 g fiber, 19 g sugars, and 1 g fat.

31. Sweet Potato Twist Smoothie:

Do you have a cold or allergies? Blend this smoothie with mango and turmeric to help relieve your symptoms and satisfy your palate! Mangos' high vitamin C content can aid in the body's defense against sickness, while turmeric may help reduce allergy symptoms like sniffles and sneezes.

Nutrition: 5 g protein, 41 g carbohydrates, 5 g fiber, 31 g sugars, and 10 g fat in 259 calories.

32: Mango-Peach Smoothie:

This smoothie is a delicious, low-calorie breakfast option that combines the flavors of sweet peaches with zesty mango. With 26 g of carbohydrates and 7 g of protein, this wholesome beverage will help you stay focused and satisfied. Because it is low in calories, we suggest having it with a slice of peanut butter toast in order to meet your macros.

Calories: about 155; protein: 7 g; fat: 3 g (1.5 g saturated); carbs: 26 g; and fiber: 3 g.

33. Smoothie with Dragon Fruit, Hibiscus, Banana, and Coconut:

Dragon fruit adds so much more to this smoothie than just a beautiful hue. Despite the high carbohydrate content, the combination of banana, coconut, and hibiscus makes this drink a high-fiber, high-magnesium meal that helps to stabilize blood pressure and blood sugar levels.

Nutrition: 21.5 g sugars (0 g added sugars), 9.5 g fat (8 g saturated fat), 222 calories, 3 g protein, 35 g carbs, and 6 g fiber.

34. Coconut Pineapple Green Smoothie:

With less than 200 calories, this smoothie is a fantastic way to boost energy during the midday hours. It's loaded with healthy ingredients, including frozen pineapple, baby spinach, and a banana. It has 30 g of carbohydrates, but just 11.5 g of sugar and 0 g of added sugar.

Nutrition: 11.5 g sugars (0 g added sugars), 7 g fat (7 g sat fat), 192 calories, 4 g protein, 30 g carbs, and 4 g fiber.

CHAPTER 9: Special Dietary Needs.

When you have cancer, your diet plays a critical role. A healthy body requires an adequate supply of calories and nutrients. However, the illness may make it difficult for you to obtain the necessities, which may vary prior to, during, and following therapy. You can also simply not feel like eating at times.

You don't have to change your diet drastically. Just a few easy tips to make healthy food tasty and simple

Prior To Treatment:

Even before your treatment starts, start making an effort to consume a nutritious diet. You have no idea what kind of adverse effects you might experience or how they will affect you. Therefore, it's a good idea to start eating healthily right away. It can support your body's continued strength and well-being.
Making plans for the days you won't feel like cooking is also a smart idea at this time.

Stock your cupboard and refrigerator with nutritious foods, particularly those that require little to no cooking.
Simple choices include
- nuts,
- applesauce,
- yogurt,
- pre-cut vegetables, and microwaveable brown rice or other nutritious grains.

Prepare large quantities of your preferred dishes and store them in the freezer.
For the first few days or weeks of your therapy, you might also wish to arrange for some friends and relatives to bring you food.
Throughout treatment, you can have days when you're not hungry and days when you wish you hadn't eaten.

Eat a lot of protein and healthy calories on your good days. This will keep your body robust and aid in healing any harm caused by your cancer or treatment.

Foods high in protein include:
- Fish eggs,
- poultry, and lean meat
- Nuts,
- seeds, and beansMilk,
- cheese, and yogurt.

Aim for a daily intake of at least 2 1/2 cups of fruits and vegetables. Add citrus fruits like oranges and grapefruits, as well as vegetables with vivid green and yellow hues. These vibrant foods are packed with beneficial minerals. Just make sure you give them a good cleaning. OriginBoost your trading abilities.

All day long, sip on plenty of liquids. Water is a wise decision. Attempt fresh-squeezed juice as well. It provides you with the liquid your body needs to stay hydrated, as well as a few extra vitamins.

Avoiding uncooked or undercooked meat, fish, and poultry is also crucial. Eat and drink no unpasteurized food or beverages.
When you're hungry, eat. If that's in the morning, have your largest meal during breakfast. If, as the day goes on, your hunger wanes, then sip meal replacements. If you find meals difficult, try eating five or six little meals throughout the day rather than two or three large ones.

Keep little, healthy snacks on hand as well. Good options include cereal, yogurt, cheese and crackers, and soup. A light lunch or supper just before a chemotherapy session may help prevent nausea.

Control Adverse Effects.

Eating enough food can be difficult due to the side effects of cancer treatments. Some of the most frequent problems may be overcome by changing your diet.
Avoid foods that are heavy in fat, grease, spice, or strong scents if you have nausea or vomiting. Every few hours, have dry things like bread or crackers. Drink clear beverages such as water, sports drinks, and broths.

Mouth or throat issues: Avoid hard foods if you have sores, soreness, or difficulty swallowing. Avert anything scratchy or abrasive, as well as spicy or acidic dishes. Eat moderately warm food—neither hot nor cold. And for drinks or soups, use a straw.

Constipation and diarrhea: It's crucial to drink plenty of water if you have diarrhea. Reduce your intake of high-fiber foods like vegetables and whole grains while increasing your fluid intake. Increase the amount of high-fiber foods in your diet gradually if you're constipated. Drinking lots of drinks is also essential for this issue.

The effects of treatment on your taste buds can be amusing. Things that you disliked previously may taste delicious today. Therefore, try new foods. Check if you enjoy tangy or sour flavors, such as those of pomegranates or ginger. Herbs like oregano, mint, and rosemary may also enhance your enjoyment of other dishes.

"Cancer Diets": Many people advertise "special" diets that they claim can either prevent cancer from returning or help treat it. Perhaps you've heard that you ought to switch to a raw diet, become a vegetarian, or go vegan. Consult your physician prior to making any significant adjustments.

Cancer cannot be cured by food. Furthermore, there is insufficient evidence to support the idea that any diet, including a vegetarian diet, can reduce the risk of cancer returning.

Maintaining a balanced diet that includes whole grains, low-fat dairy, fruits, vegetables, lean proteins, and other nutrients is your best option. Reduce your intake of alcohol, sugar, coffee, and salt.

Thanks For Reading And More Importantly, Thanks For Getting Back This Book.